How to Banish Worry &
Live a Panic-Free Life

The ANTI ANXIETY

Formula

<u>**Disclaimer Notice:**</u>

Please note the information contained within this document is for educational and entertainment purposes only. Every attempt has been made to provide accurate, up to date and reliable complete information. No warranties of any kind are expressed or implied. Readers acknowledge that the author is not engaging in the rendering of legal, financial, medical or professional advice.

By reading this document, the reader agrees that under no circumstances are we responsible for any losses, direct or indirect, which are incurred as a result of the use of information contained within this document, including, but not limited to, — errors, omissions, or inaccuracies.

TABLE OF CONTENTS

Introduction 7

Chapter 1 - You and Your Anxiety: How to Overcome Your Stuck Points 10

The Multifaceted You 11

Worksheet 1 - What Do You See? 11

Understanding Your Anxiety and What It Is Doing to You 12

Worksheet 2 - What Does Your Behavior Say of You? 13

Reflecting upon Your Triggers and Identifying Beliefs That are Standing in Your Way 14

Worksheet 3 - Imagery Exposure 15

Mindfully Moving Beyond the Beliefs Blocking Your Path 17

Worksheet 4 - Recognizing Your Challenges 18

Where to Next? 19

Chapter 2 - Your Mind, Your Body: How to Face Your Inner Demons 21

Putting Events, Emotions, and Vibrations Together 21

Imagining the Worst 23

Self-Blame. Self Loathe. All of it 24

Connecting Them with Your Mind and Body 27

Worksheet 7 - Talking Yourself Out of Anxiety 28

Chapter 3 - Overcoming Resistance to Change 31

Recognizing Any Resistance to Change 31

Worksheet 8 – The Fear of Change Quiz 32

Belief-Systems That Stop You from Acting on a Change 33

Self-Sympathy. Self-Loathe. Anxiety. Depression...........................33

What Do You See?..34

Worksheet 9 - Acting on Your Change -Blocking Systems...............35

Re-writing Your Life - One Change at a Time 35

Chapter 4 – Reflection: How to Arrive at Acceptance and Move on From There 40

Understanding Your Body Signals 41

Worksheet 10 - Tracking Your Body's Signals 42

Minding Your Moods 43

Worksheet 11 - Mood Tracker 44

Finding Acceptance..46

What Are Distorted Thought Patterns?...................................46

Worksheet 12 - Distorted Thoughts Tracker 49

Assessing Your Present and Preparing a Plan for the Future 50

Connect with Now 51

Worksheet 13 - Setting Goals 51

Chapter 5 - Acting against Angst: How to Act on Your Fears and Achieve Your Goals 53

Evading Avoidance...53

Worksheet 14 - Identifying Your Fears 54

Acting against Your Fears 55

Worksheet 15 - Taking the Step-Up Approach 56

Begin the Process 57

Create and Execute Your Plan...57

Consider Every Aspect That Might Influence, Conflict or Jeopardize Your Plan..58

Be Mindful of Any possible Setbacks, But Don't Let Them Wear You Down 59

No Need to Hurry...59

Know When You've Tried Too Long.......................................60

It's Okay to Fall. Fail Too..60

Realign Your Plan. Improvise Too...60

Complete What You've Taken 61

Become a Better Version of You 62

Chapter 6 - Navigating Self-Imposed Obstacles: How to Stop

Being a Hard Task Master **64**

Moving Ahead of Any past Pain Memories 65

Moving Away from the Past You Need to Leave Behind 67

Worksheet 17 - Letting Go 67

Overcoming Obsessions 68

Worksheet 18 - Recognizing Any Obsessions 69

New Beginnings 71

Worksheet 20 – Creating Tomorrow 72

Chapter 7 - Preventing Burnout: How to Overcome Your Anxiety without Getting Tied-Down by the Idea of Perfection 75

Setting Real Expectations 75

Worksheet 21 – Expectation Tracker 76

Perfectionism and Borrowed Expectations 78

Leaving No Room to Pause. Falter Too 78

Avoiding Comparisons 79

Worksheet 22 - Becoming the Change You Want to See 79

Change Everything If You Have To, but Change Them One Thing at a Time 80

Fear of Feedback...80

Worksheet 23 - Overcoming Feedback Fears 81

Reward Yourself. You've Made Great Progress 82

Chapter 8 - You've Got This: How to Banish Worry and Live Panic-Free..**85**

Simplify 86

Breathe 86

Exercise 87

Express Yourself. Talk It Out or Journal Your Thoughts 88

Listen to Music..89

Spend Time with Pets 90

Give Your Mind Something More Productive to Chew On 90

Stay in the Present 91

You Decide. Ready or Not? 92

Worksheet 24 - Gathering Your Tools 92

Conclusion **93**

Introduction

Do any of these statements sound familiar?

You worry too much.

You must drag yourself out of the bed every morning and often wake up feeling sad for no obvious reason.

You're disposed to making negative predictions.

You worry about the worst that could happen in any situation.

You take negative feedback very personally.

You're your biggest critic.

You avoid people more than you should.

Anything less than perfection feels like failure.

If they do, then there's a chance that you're experiencing some degree of anxiety and/or depression. Unpleasant feelings are a part of our daily lives. They are there to teach us a lesson. Once we've learned our lesson, they often move on, but might come back with another lesson later.

As a result of these experiences, you're likely to feel sad and stressed. These are perfectly normal emotions to go through from time to time. Everyone feels low and apprehensive about something or the other at some point in their lives. But when these unpleasant emotions begin to consume you, then you must act before it's too late.

Fortunately, these feelings can be healed. They can be made to shift to a more positive and constructive space. And we are here to help. The *Anti-Anxiety Formula* book has been written with especially this in mind.

You will find a wide range of skills and tools to help manage and overcome your anxiety. This book is filled with questions that help you reflect and find answers for yourself. We urge you to give every practice a try before deciding on the ones that work best for you.

On that note, we welcome you to our book titled, '*The Anti-Anxiety Formula*.' We've had an enriching time creating this book and hope that experience translates to our readers too.

YOU AND YOUR ANXIETY

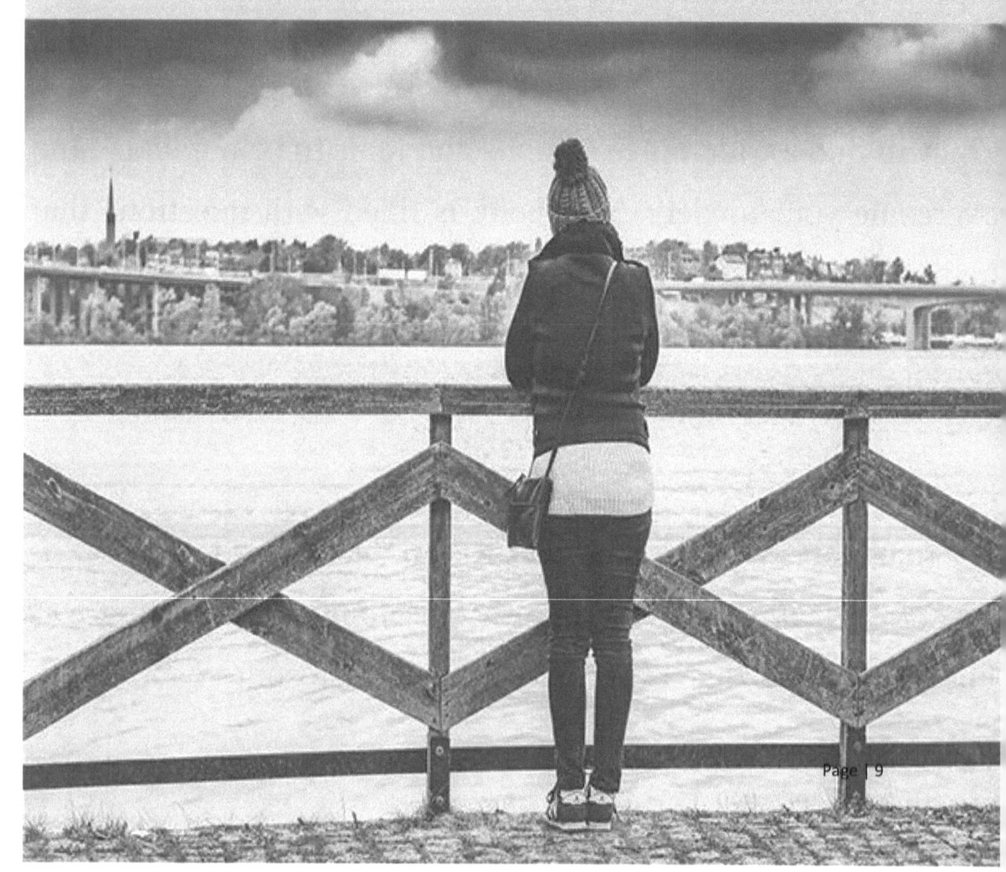

Chapter 1 - You and Your Anxiety: How to Overcome Your Stuck Points

Anxiety can creep up on you in many ways from physical and behavioral symptoms that are obvious to subtler symptoms that mess with your emotional and cognitive state of being. Yet, each time, it can leave behind a somewhat similar and familiar feeling - the feeling of being a little more lost, battered, and alone.

No anxious person has the same set of symptoms, which is why each person's anxiety is unique and therefore their individual journey. That said, most people have some of each type of the symptoms, only in different combinations, which makes understanding how it works more appreciable. This chapter focuses on personality concepts that will help you understand how your anxiety works.

The Multifaceted You

Now, you cannot understand the average anxious person to understand your anxiety. You don't need to either. You need to understand the many dimensions within which you and your anxiety exist. Once you start identifying these dimensions which are mostly characterized by triggers and symptoms, you'll be able to work around them, and in time, overcome them too.

Worksheet 1 - What Do You See?

Here's a quick worksheet for you. Do any of these situations sound familiar to you?

- You dislike change. Every time you are put into a new situation, you feel restless and worried.
- You over process information, decisions, and possibilities before acting.
- You tend to be pessimistic about the present and future.
- You constantly dwell into negative past experiences.
- You worry about everything.
- You feel awkward when someone compliments you. You also believe they don't mean their compliments or are mocking you in some way.

- You are your harshest critic.

While there is no scoring system here to rate your anxiety, it does help you to understand if you are anxiety-prone or not. The more items you check, the more likely you are suffering from anxiety, depression or both.

Understanding Your Anxiety and What It Is Doing to You

Anxiety on the inside can affect what you do and how you act on the outside. And so, if you were to observe your mind and body carefully, you might be able to notice some signs, behavioral and physical, that can tell you what your anxiety might be doing to you. For instance, an anxious person might be dealing with several conflicting and apprehensive thoughts. The internal noise and fear that reverberates inside might make them appear tired, withdrawn, and/or nervous.

Worksheet 2 - What Does Your Behavior Say of You?

Check off statements that apply to you.

- I find myself crying for no reason.
- There are times when I feel empty and can't make myself do what I want to do.
- I avoid socializing.
- I avoid risks.
- I also avoid doing fun stuff because I worry about the possible risk involved.
- I'm afraid of failure and judgment.
- I get fidgety.
- I obsess over the past, worry about the future, and can rarely stay in the present.

And About Your Body?

- I have no appetite.
- I'm always hungry.
- My palms sweat all the time.
- I can feel nauseous, lightheaded, cold, and shaky when anxious.
- My heart races when I worry.

- I feel cold and weak too.
- I have very little energy.

Again, there is no scoring system to rate your anxiety. The more symptoms you check off, the more likely you are experiencing anxiety.

Note: Now, some of the above symptoms can also result from various other reasons, and so, we suggest you consult your primary care physician before making any conclusions.

Reflecting upon Your Triggers and Identifying Beliefs That are Standing in Your Way

If you could follow an anxious mind, you might see patterns of unfavorable thoughts that keep playing on and off. These thoughts might be triggers to the anxiety itself, and so addressing them is very important. A clinical technique called imagery exposure, used in therapy, can help address the triggers as well as identify their sources.

Worksheet 3 - Imagery Exposure

Sit with yourself and truthfully reflect on any unfavorable thoughts that play in your mind, the thoughts that stop you from concentrating and being in the present, the ones that you want to forget, but cannot, and the ones that you might have kept buried and might not necessarily like to share with others. You can also reflect on any worry thoughts, the ones that haven't happened yet, but you fear.

Recall the sights and sounds of the situation as if it were happening in front of you, as we speak, in as much detail as you can. Bring the image of the embarrassment, avoidance, worry, fear, hurt, and/or guilt vividly to mind. Deliberate on the image, living the experience thoroughly once.

Let the thoughts stay with you until they decide to leave you at their will. Repeat this exercise once every day for as long as you want. As you progress further, you'll begin to see reasons. You'll realize beliefs that have been blocking your path - your stuck points so to speak. You'll find solutions to overcome the negative outcomes of your triggers. Finally, you'll find peace.

This Is the Start

Now, this is a gradual process and is the first step to addressing your anxiety. Once you know what's causing your anxiety, you can, in time, find ways to manage or overcome it (and this book shows you exactly how to do that.)

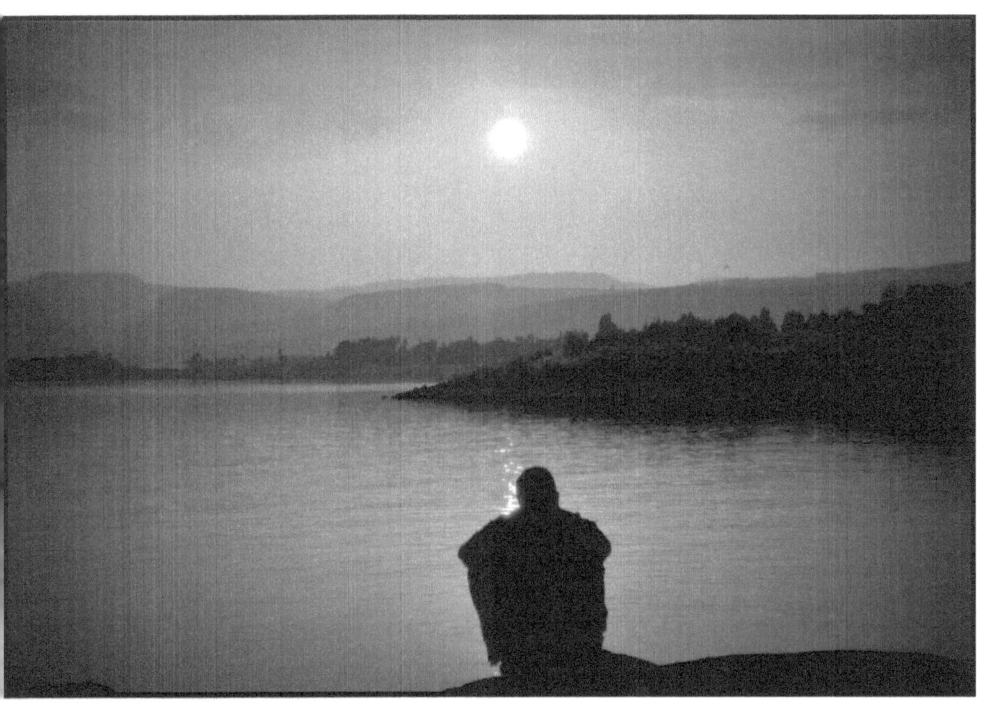

Mindfully Moving Beyond the Beliefs Blocking Your Path

The thing about stuck points is that when we're caught in one, we don't often think about ways to work around them and move forward. We don't shift into problem-solving mode and weigh our options (mostly because we don't know how to and therefore cannot).

To be able to solve problems, you must think realistically, coherently, without any chatter. And unfortunately, when anxious, our mind can get tied up in its contemplation wheel and fail to work on more productive and purposeful things.

For instance, imagine you have a team deadline to meet, but a member of your team isn't contributing equally. Instead of working yourself up about why he/she isn't doing their bit, it would be more useful to think about ways to help them step up or help reach the immediate deadline.

So, you can:
- Speak to the member and let them know where they need to step up, while suggesting some options to work things out.
- Give them simpler jobs or a checklist to do every day.

- Split the work amongst others in the team.
- Get the job done first and then look at a more permanent way out.

Mindfully forcing yourself to look at the possible solutions as opposed to mulling on the problem can help relieve the stress of rumination. Focusing on a constructive solution will shift you to a more positive state of mind just as achieving the solution will shift you to a state of peace and contentment.

Worksheet 4 - Recognizing Your Challenges

- Reflect on the one stuck point that is stopping you from moving forward.
- Define your best three realistic solutions. Keep them simple and achievable.
- Decide what you need to act on them.
- Decide how long you need to gather these tools.
- Start working towards these goals.

Where to Next?

At this point, you should pat yourself on the back. You've made progress and are a step closer to understanding and managing your anxiety. The next few chapters discuss aspects that go a little beyond your thoughts. It dwells on areas such as your mind and your body and their role in your anxiety. Take a moment to pause now and then. Stay in the present. This is your reality. Where do you want to be?

Ok, let's start preparing for your future.

2

YOUR MIND, YOUR BODY

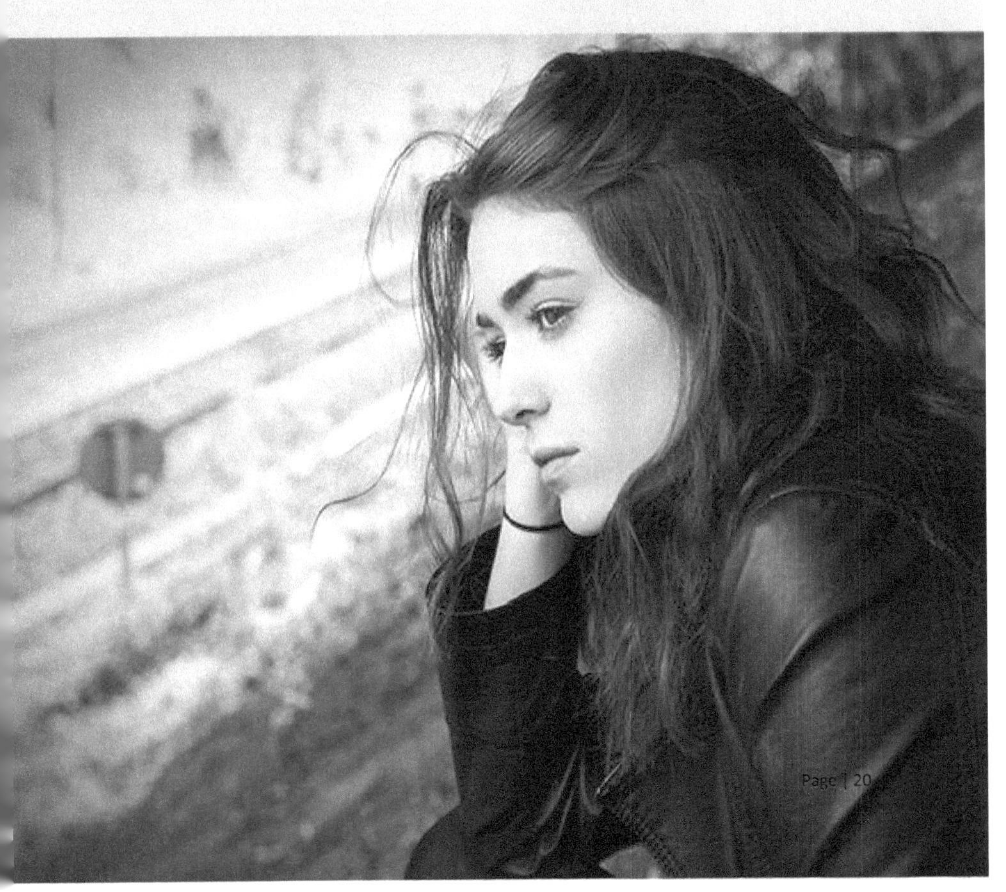

Chapter 2 - Your Mind, Your Body: How to Face Your Inner Demons

If you're reading this book, you probably experience anxiety in one form or the other, but don't know where those feelings come from. This is completely normal and is a sign that you are ready-ready to understand the origins of your anxiety and ready to work your way around and overcome it. This chapter shows you how to address your mental and physical battles while digging deeper into the source of your anxiety - your inner demons so to speak.

Putting Events, Emotions, and Vibrations Together

The confusion and anxiety you feel today could be the result of seeds planted in your past. And so, dwelling into your past, into memories that you perhaps would otherwise like to avoid and forget or have consciously erased from your mind, can help piece together the source of your anxiety.

Disclaimer: Some of the memories you revisit through the questions put forth in this book may evoke unexpected reactions and that's completely normal. You may feel slightly uncomfortable and that's normal too. As unexpected and unpleasant as they can be, they are important as they may lead you to the origins of your problems. That said, if you become overtly overwhelmed, you may stop the exercise and seek professional help. We recommend you also have someone who can have your back.

Worksheet 5 - Review Your World

Many times, people with anxiety know they are experiencing anxious feelings. They can tell you how they feel, but don't know why they feel a way. That's why journaling can be such an important tool to help address and overcome anxiety.

- Daily, for two weeks at least, mindfully observe your thoughts, emotions, and bodily reactions.

- Ask yourself what is going on when you start noticing your emotions and body signals. Write your experiences when they are fresh.

- Use feeling words to describe any powerful and/or repetitive emotion. For instance, happy, energetic, nervous, sweaty, tired, dizzy and so on.

- Because we want to know the cause of your anxiety, especially note down the feelings that make you feel anxious. Make a note of the situations that led up to it.

- At the end of the second week (or more if you wish), reflect on the anxious feelings and situations. Compare them to your notes from worksheet 4. Do you see a pattern? Make a note of your thoughts.

Imagining the Worst

Life can be rough sometimes. Bad things can happen without a plan and then can leave behind a sense of lasting pain and fear. But sometimes, our mind can fantasize about things that never happened and probably might never happen too. These things can be our biggest fears. We can imagine catastrophic events and jump to the worst possible conclusions with no reason or logic. And so, by doing that repeatedly, you live the experience that many times (because your mind and body might not be able to differentiate real from the imaginary world).

Self-Blame. Self Loathe. All of it.

Rachel suffers from constant worry and anxiety. Some she says are the result of the busy life she leads. She wakes up at 5 am every day, travels an hour to reach work, is constantly rushing through meetings and deadlines, takes another hour to reach home at 8 pm, cooks and finishes her dinner, prepares for the next day before she can go to sleep at 11 pm.

Sometimes things get rough, her anxiety kicks in as a result of her worst imagination. Here's how she says her mind plays out events when that happens: As a result, she blames and hates herself.

My throat hurts. I think I can feel a bump. What if it's cancer? Am I going to die? What will happen to my family once I'm gone? Will they miss me?

I remember a bad/traumatic experience and replay that even repeatedly, imagining it is happening again. Sometimes, I imagine it being worse too and my responses are very real.

I see a group of people giggling in front of me. Are they laughing at me? Is it my dress? Do I look okay? Did I do something odd or funny? I need to get out of here. Why do people always make fun of me? I don't deserve this. Nobody likes me. I'm hopeless.

My manager didn't greet me as usual. I wonder if he/she is upset about my work. What if I get fired? What about my bills? Why can't I do anything right? Why am I never good enough? I hate myself.

Worksheet 6 - Living Your Biggest Fears - This Time with Reason

Decide to live your biggest fears once again-this time more mindfully. Take one fear at a time and if there are many, then move over to the next fear only after you've completely made peace with the previous one. Sure, this might take time, but the positive effects can last a lifetime. So, don't rush. Again, decide whether you want to have someone around to watch your back.

Sit with yourself when you're feeling most secure and comfortable. Remind yourself that what you are going to experience isn't real. Remind yourself to disconnect from emotional trauma you are knowingly going to put yourself through. Remind yourself of the purpose of this exercise. You want to dig deeper into your fears and understand what you are learning from it is. Once you recognize this, you can work on the learning and the suffering will gradually decrease.

And when you're ready, go through the experience, your biggest fears, the worse possible situations, your inner demons so to speak. What is it that keeps troubling you? Why do you keep inviting this experience into your life? Is there a lesson?

What's the worst possible? Okay that happened. Can it get worse? Imagine that too. Live the experience all the time telling yourself that this isn't real and isn't happening now.

Again, when you're ready, bring yourself back to the present and reflect on your thoughts and emotions. Write them down when you are ready.

Repeat this exercise whenever you are ready for it and until the time you've made peace with the fear and can move on.

The best way to gain perspective is to mindfully talk to yourself as you experience the rush of fantasized images. Now that you know that that can happen, the next time you catch yourself doing something like that, tell yourself:

- This isn't real and it's not happening now
- Whatever happens, I can cope
- I am going to stop causing my suffering
- I am doing great. I've got this
- I love myself. I feel great.

Connecting Them with Your Mind and Body

Remember, you can manage and even overcome your anxiety by learning to feel better with introspection. Ask yourself as many questions about your anxiety. Persist because deep down, you have and know the answers. Observe your relationship with your feelings, thoughts and your body's responses to them. Track them and talk yourself to a better, calmer, and panic-free state of mind. Yes, you can!

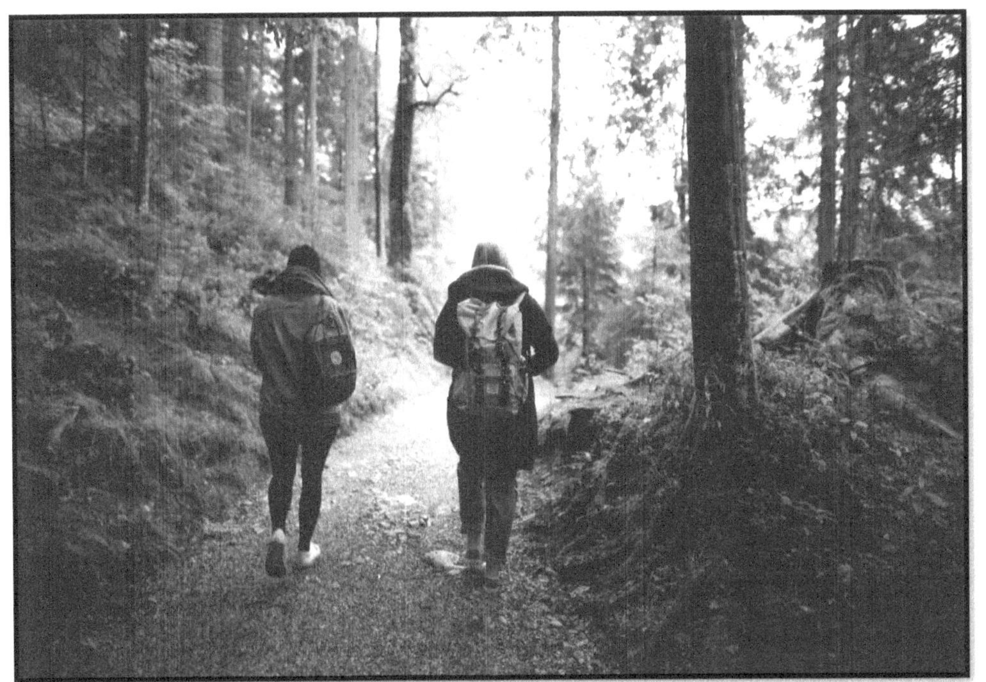

Worksheet 7 - Talking Yourself Out of Anxiety

- Each day, record events that made you anxious. Elaborate and specify the event as well as your thoughts and bodily reactions to it.
- Use feeling words to describe your emotions.
- Go through the experience and decide to make peace with it. Keep telling yourself that the present is great, and the future will be even better.

- Work on your feelings. Talk to yourself. Gather support from others if you want to.

- At the end of every week, look back on your tracker and evaluate your progress.

- How are you feeling?

As you work through the exercises presented this book, you should become more aware of your anxiety, the reasons for it as well as how your body reacts to events in your life. The more knowledge you gain, the better you can understand and manage your anxiety. So, keep at it.

3

OVERCOMING RESISTANCE TO CHANGE

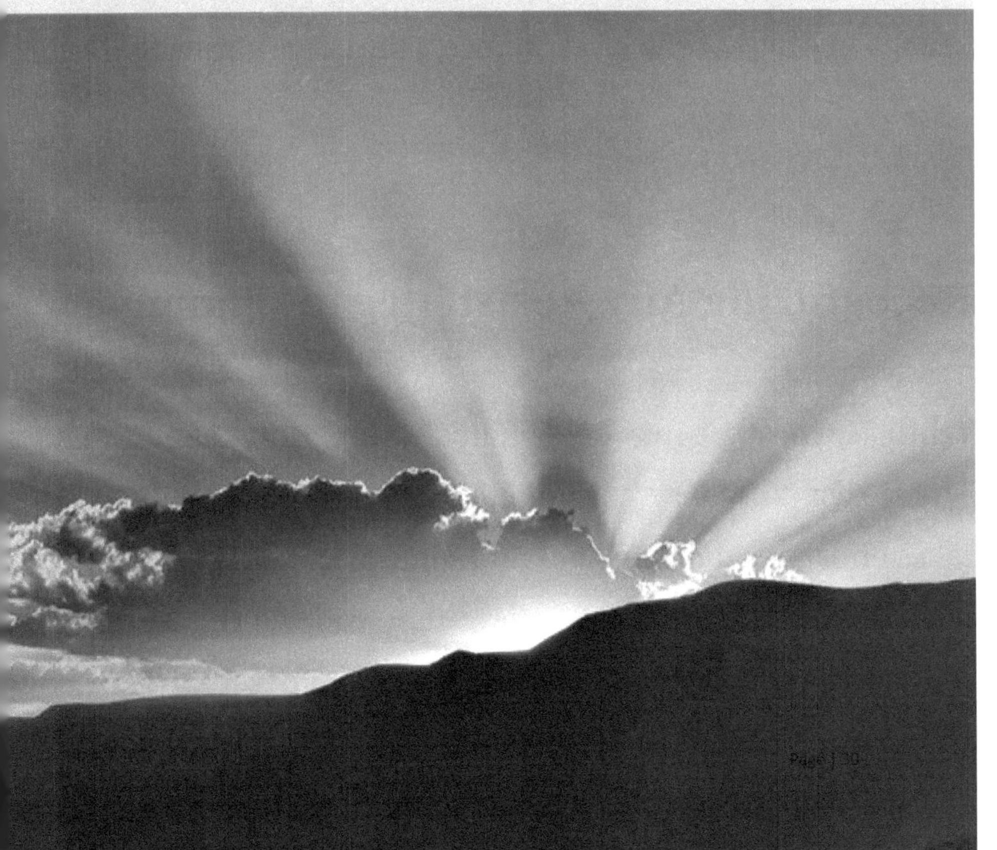

Chapter 3 - Overcoming Resistance to Change

Being watchful, precautious and reflective while taking your time to do important things might have their advantages, but if your habit is inching more towards procrastination, then it could be that you are resistant to change. And frankly speaking, you are not alone. Most people, in some way or the other, are resistant to change because of the level of uncertainty it brings with it.

Recognizing Any Resistance to Change

Truth is, most people hold many assumptions about change. They resist it because it is unknown and therefore frightening. It takes effort to act on changes and some aren't so keen on putting in that effort. Some don't believe they can see the results they seek and so why try? Others think they don't deserve to be happy and so don't change to improve their situations. Some get so lost and stuck up in the cycle of anxiety that they fail to recognize the scope for change, for a better life. While most of these thoughts are indeed assumptions, they can become the very beliefs that stand in the way of what you want to achieve.

Take the quiz below to know if you are resistant to change

Worksheet 8 – The Fear of Change Quiz

Check the statements that resonate with your feelings.

- I can take a risk, but what if I fail? Maybe, I should not.
- I can seek help, but what if no one offers? What if I get rejected?
- I always have trouble acting on changes, what if I mess up again?
- What's the point? I always get my hopes up but fail and get disappointed.
- I can't do this. I'll never change. Why try? I don't want to fail again.
- I'm too anxious to succeed.

Belief-Systems That Stop You from Acting on a Change

- It's better to be realistic and accept my shortcomings. I'm not going to change. I know that.
- I'm not as good as the others. Surely, I can't compete with them.
- I don't want to ask for help. It will make my weaknesses obvious and then everyone will know.
- I don't think anyone cares. No one will help me.
- I messed up when I could have made things better. That was my only chance. I can't do anything now and must settle for what comes my way.

Self-Sympathy.   Self-Loathe.   Anxiety. Depression.

- I am helpless. No one cares and no one will help
- I've been misunderstood and mistreated all my life. No one changed for me. So why should I change?
- They don't realize that I don't like being this way, that I have no choice.

- This is so unfair
- Oh, forget it. I'm hopeless. I hate myself.
- People will mock me. They already are. I know it and I want to hide.
- There is no point. I can't see any purpose in my life.
- I'm so alone and I want to cry

What Do You See?

The more checks you have, the more you are resistant to change. While the above statements might not be pleasant to realize about oneself, it isn't entirely your fault if you hold any or many of these blocking beliefs.

People pick these ideas as a result of the circumstances and experiences they've lived. What's important is that you can change, we all can. You can change right now, or you can try and fail and try again. Both are normal and positive outcomes. Keep at it because the harder you try and the more you persist, the more likely you're going to become the change.

Worksheet 9 - Acting on Your Change - Blocking Systems

- From the statements checked off above, write down each of your change-clocking beliefs.
- Write down their justifications. Why do you do them? Introspect and elaborate.
- What are the advantages of changing that belief? What are the disadvantages too?
- Weigh them. What scores higher?
- Are your beliefs causing you more harm than good?
- What's stopping you from embracing the change?
- Make a list of small actions to reach the bigger change you seek.
- Work on consistency first. Force yourself to do one action at a time, completely. Do it every time.
- The more you work on your consistency, the more habitualized your routine will become.

Re-writing Your Life - One Change at a Time

Our minds are capable of wonderful things. They can envision a beautiful life. They can create stories, piece together minute details that together give the story the ending it needs. Use this to advantage. Talk to your mind. Listen to it too. Establish a relationship with it and once it feels heard and starts responding, teach it to create positive and inspirational thoughts for you.

Plant the seeds to begin the story. For instance, you want to work on your fitness and want to start a jogging routine every morning. Imagine yourself doing this every day. Imagine your life just as you want it to be.

Remember to be realistic in your narrative, so keep the struggles too because when you do, you give your mind a heads-up of what might come its way. Think about the success you are going to achieve. Imagine and feel it too. These images are powerful building blocks. They can then be picked up by your mind to build and breathe life. As they say, you dream, and you become.

Steve has always had troubling embracing change. He works in a multinational company but has been stuck in the same position for the past 15 years. It's not like he doesn't want a change. He craves for change in his job. He wants to do something new. But he is unwilling to learn and adapt to new methods. As a result, he does what he is told to do and nothing more. Most colleagues his age have jumped a couple or more positions. It does bother him, but he believes he can't do anything about it. He struggles to stay focused and interested at work and hence isn't as effective as the others.

His peers are younger, and he thinks that's why they turn out smarter. He also thinks they secretly make fun of him. His batch mates are way up in the ladder to socialize with anymore (or so he thinks), and he doesn't make efforts to mingle with the younger lads too. As a result of all this, his anxiety has taken an ugly turn.

He's anxious all the time. Fortunately, an old friend notices Steve's behavior and reaches out to him. He tells him about his resistance to change and how that is stopping him from becoming a better version of himself. Because Steve is at a point when he really wants to change, he listens. He decides to give change a shot. He makes plans and decides to act on them, one change at a time. He also reaches out to his family and other friends for support. They all want to help and do their best to keep him motivated.

Two years down the line, Steve is a complexly transformed person. He works harder and smarter and even mingles with all his colleagues. He's made plenty of new friends and enjoys his weekends with family.

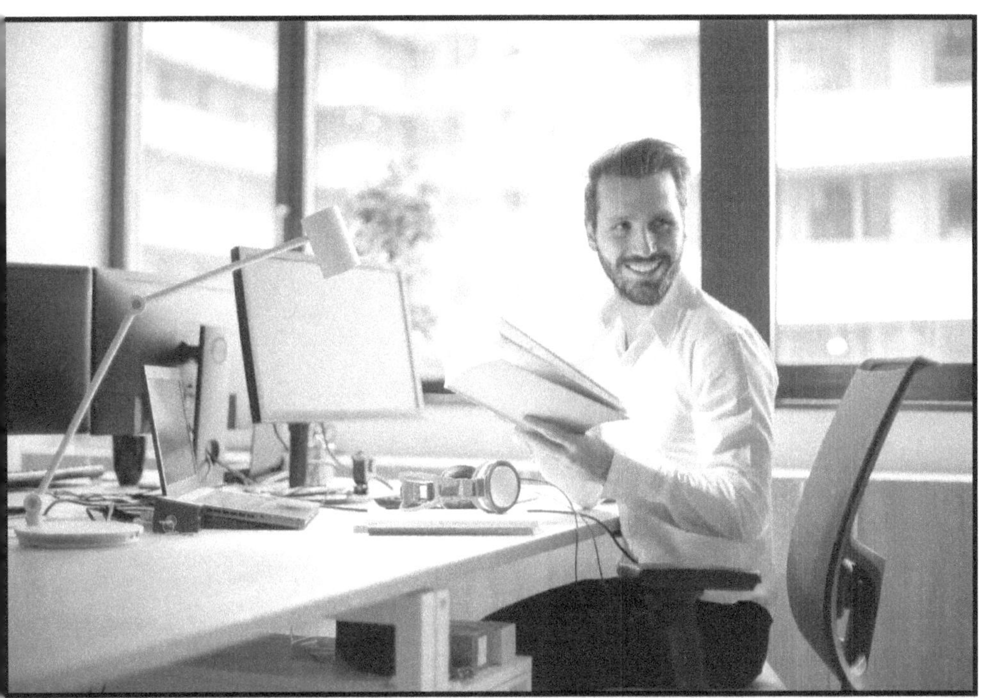

He's going to complete his masters from a prestigious university and is looking forward to the new prospects that will bring him. Steve is happy. He hardly feels anxious anymore and when he does, he knows how to stay on top of it. His family and friends are happy for Steve and love spending time with him.

Well, like Steve, you too can rewrite your current life script. You can become the change you always wanted to be.

The time is NOW.

4

REFLECTION

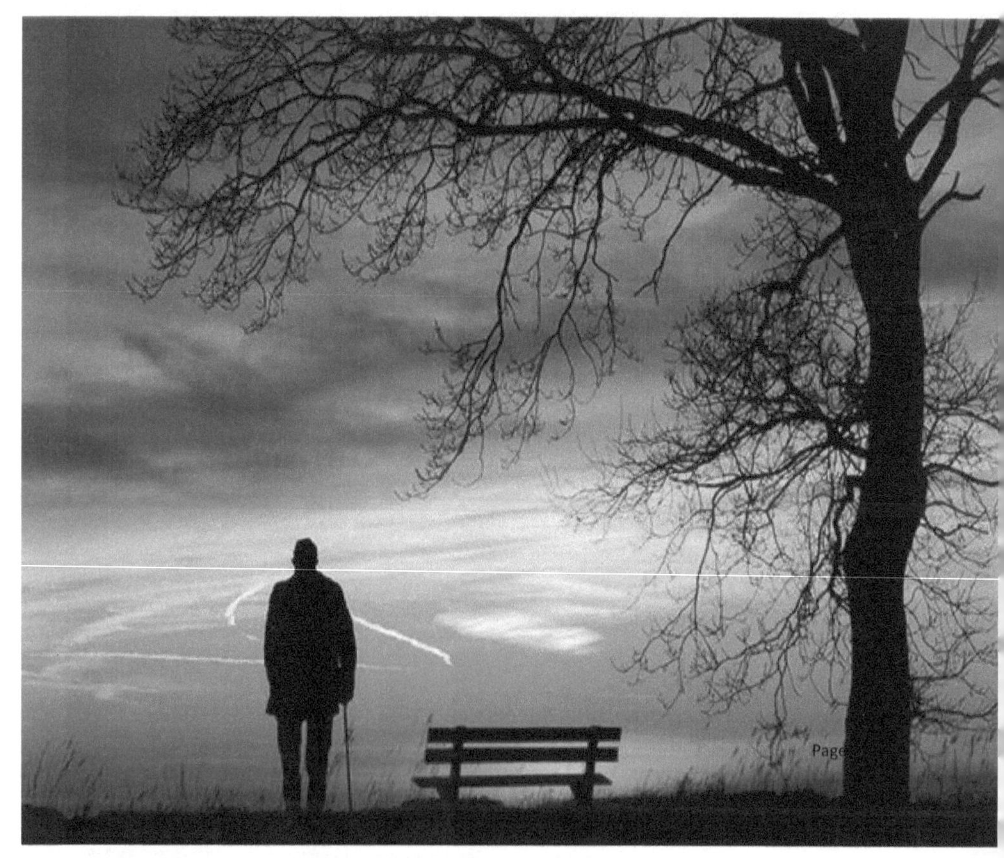

Chapter 4 – Reflection: How to Arrive at Acceptance and Move on From There

Managing and overcoming anxiety takes work, a lot of work through self-observation and introspection, which is why this book is filled with worksheets that help you ask the right questions and as a result find the right answers.

This process isn't easy. It isn't quick too. But we guarantee that the rewards are long-lasting and worthy. In this chapter, we speak about reaching a place where you can accept your current situation and plan. We provide guidelines that help you reflect and reassess your situation, the reasons for it, and ways to manage it too.

The first step to this process is to monitor your body's responses to events that bring on your anxiety. This step is vital because sometimes, people don't realize they're going through an anxiety attack until they begin to experience some physical components of it.

Once you are physically aware of what your body is going through, you can track your feelings and observe their relationship with each other. Finally, we show you how to become more aware of your present state of mind. We show you how to accept it and move on from there.

Understanding Your Body Signals

Daisy is a bit taken aback when her doctor diagnoses her with anxiety. Her doctor suggests she spend more time listening to her body and so she tries to understand her body signals by writing down unpleasant physical sensations as she experiences them. What she discovers over a week surprises her. She realizes she is experiencing some of the tell-tale signs of anxiety. She decides to take control of it and with the guidance of her doctor starts tuning in to find a way out of her dilemma.

Worksheet 10 - Tracking Your Body's Signals

Here is a list of common bodily symptoms and signs of anxiety. Keep a track of any signs you experience for a week, along with the day you experienced it and the situation that led up to the experience. Now, some of the symptoms might be like that of an illness. If your symptoms are indicative of an illness, then consult your doctor for advice. But if your symptoms are a result of your anxiety, then you're likely to have an emotional thought that led to it.

- Increased heart rate
- Difficulty in breathing
- Stomach discomfort
- Headache
- Dizziness
- Sweaty hands, palms, feet, forehead
- Light-headedness
- Tightening of chest
- Feeling disoriented
- Feeling nauseous
- Feeling lonely and sad

At the end of each day, review your notes. Take time to think about what you feel. Write your feelings.

Minding Your Moods

After you become more aware of your body's signals, you might be able to connect them with your changing moods.

Track your moods every day for a week. How do you feel when you are happy? How do you feel when you think you are feeling anxious? What is your mood like? How do you react to emotional situations? Can you identify it as you experience it? What are your thoughts at such a time? How much control do you have over your thoughts and responses, your moods too?

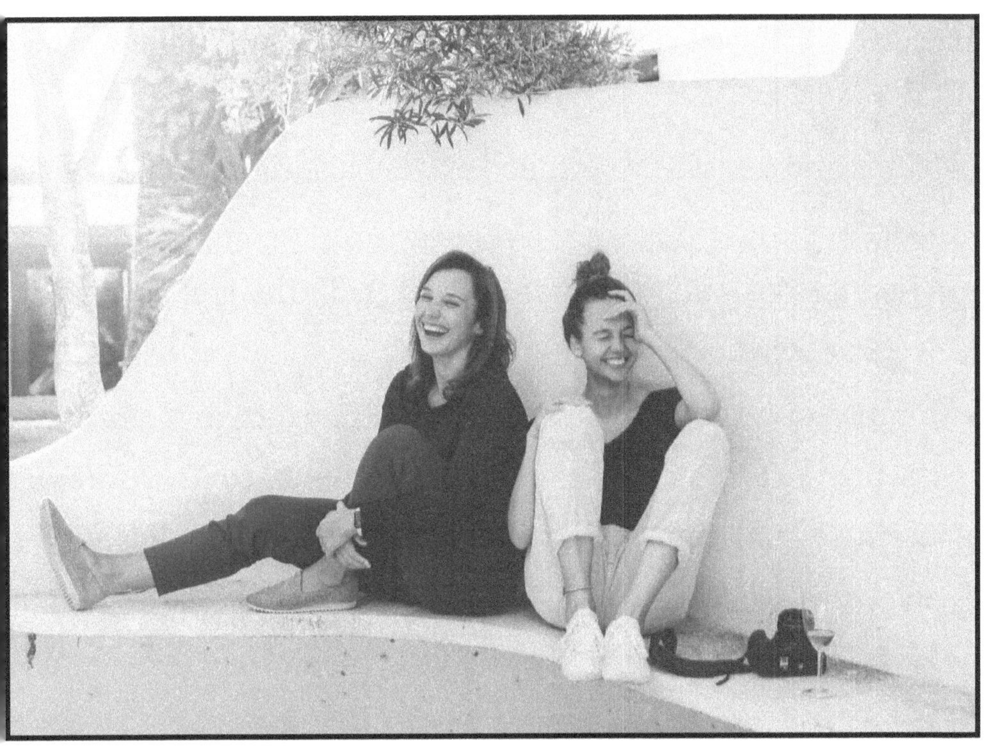

Worksheet 11 - Mood Tracker

- Each day, circle all the feeling words mentioned below that describe your emotions.

Sadness	Fear	Shame	Anger
Downhearted	Frightened	Guilty	Hostile
Defeated	Edgy	Apologetic	Violent
Forlorn	Troubled	Self-Conscious	Resentful
Discouraged	Reserved	Shunned	Annoyed

| Dejected | Alarmed | Dishonored | Irritable |

- Think and describe your mood and behavioral patterns at such times.
- Describe the situations that led to it. Your thoughts when you were experiencing it.
- Simply observe and describe your thoughts and reactions during the first week. Try and yield a level of control over any negative and unpleasant thoughts and moods during the second week.
- How are you feeling? Where are you now? Where do you want to be?
- Continue to balance your thoughts and mood swings. Do you see any progress?
- Where are you now? Where do you want to be?

Rehabilitating Your Thoughts

Now that you've spent a little time with your mind and body, you might have a fair idea of what they're trying to tell you. This understanding will only get deeper and more intuitive as you understand yourself and your anxiety better (and you'll get there as you keep working on the worksheets).

Finding Acceptance

Now, it's time to move on to the phase of acceptance. And to get there, you must first unearth and remove any distorted thought patterns that might be stopping you from moving on.

What Are Distorted Thought Patterns?

Distorted thoughts are thoughts that are disconnected and different from reality. They are thoughts you tell yourself to avoid reality. Here are some examples of distorted thought patterns.

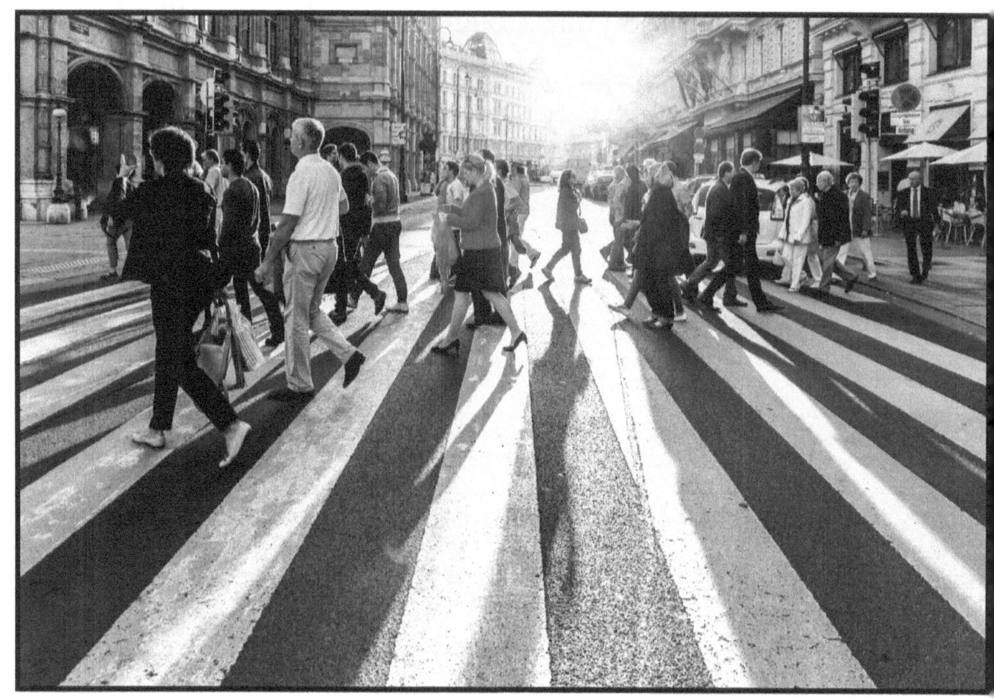

Expanding and shrinking: Your mind exaggerates the unpleasantness of the task on hand and underestimates your reluctance and/or incapability of doing it.

For instance, you may think, "It's impossible to solve this problem. Nobody can do it. Truth is, a few people in your team might have been able to do it. You dismiss it as impossible and therefore don't try and seek assistance.

Filtering: Your mind filters out information and feedback to its inconvenience. For instance, you receive feedback on your performance. You have three good scores and two poor ones. Your mind can filter this either way. It can make you believe that you were good in three and so the other two don't matter or it can make you ignore the three and focus on how miserable you are.

Dismissing evidence: Your mind discards evidence that may challenge its negative narrative. For instance, you are preparing for an exam and are worried that the lessons you skipped might end up in the paper. And so, your mind dismisses it by believing it already knows that those lessons will be ignored.

Generalizing: You look at a single, unpleasant incidence and decide that that event represents a general, unrelenting trend. For instance, you tell your friends that they are never there for you and are always late when they might have missed a few events and are caring and punctual people.

Presumptuous: You assume that you know what others are thinking without confirming it with them. For instance, you take it for granted that the other person might be ok with your choice of decisions for them.

Emotional Reasoning: If you're feeling something, then that is the truth, the reality. For instance, if you're afraid of something, then it must be dangerous for you. If you don't like working on your anxiety, then you believe that you cannot overcome it and therefore must settle with it.

Unreliable forecasting: You assume a negative thought will manifest into reality. You fear driving and so you convince yourself that you're likely to meet with an accident if you drive.

Overcoming Any Distorted Thought Patterns

Worksheet 12 - Distorted Thoughts Tracker

- Reflect on the above table. Take time to truly reflect on each pattern. And when you are open and ready, spend time to check if you display any of them. You can also ask a close friend/relative to give you their honest opinion.
- Once you identify a pattern, mindfully try and avoid this every time you catch yourself falling into the trend. Again, seek assistance from loved ones if you can.
- Tracking your thoughts and looking for distortions in them helps put things in better perspective, which in turn starts

improving your mood and reduces anxiety. So, stay honest and patient.

Assessing Your Present and Preparing a Plan for the Future

Now that you know your pitfalls and the stuck points that are stopping you from moving ahead, accept them, without guilt or resentment (it makes the process of letting go of them easier). Face your problems and take action to change it. Assess your responsibility and determine your next steps. Start by:

- Replacing any negative thoughts with positive and constructive thoughts
- Change your perspective. Become more aware- of yourself and your surroundings, of the reality too.
- Stay honest and open to feedback and change
- Distinguish the past from the present
- Take direct action against problematic thoughts

Connect with Now

Ask yourself:

- Where are you now?
- Where do you want to be?

Worksheet 13 - Setting Goals

- Can you think of anything that you want more than you fear? Your example could be anything from investing in a property, becoming more fit, creating stronger social ties. Or it can be facing your fear itself.
- If you can't think of anything right now, don't rush through. Take time to let the question marinate for a few days, weeks, even months perhaps.
- Keep going back to it to see if you have something that aligns with your purpose in life.
- Write them down when they hit you (and they will).

Great! Now you have your goals in front of you. What can stop you from achieving them?

Nothing! The next few chapters will show you how.

ACTION AGAINST
ANGST

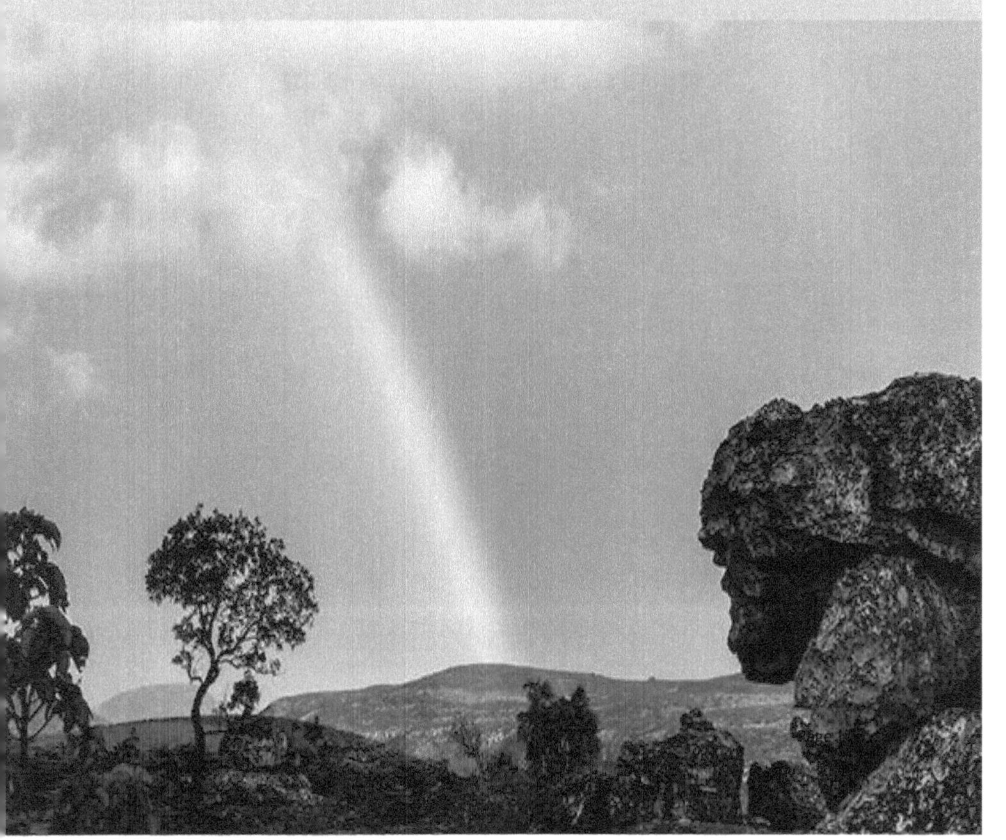

Chapter 5 - Acting against Angst: How to Act on Your Fears and Achieve Your Goals

If introspection and mindfulness can help you understand the origins and outcomes of your anxiety, changing your behavior can help you overcome it. The previous chapters showed you how to arrive at your goals. They showed you a glimpse of what you can be. This chapter shows you how you can have that experience for a lifetime. By setting goals, you can change your narrative. And by changing what you do, you can change the way you feel.

Evading Avoidance

If you experience fear and anxiety, you probably avoid the things that make you feel uncomfortable. For instance, if you don't like crowds or if socializing makes you feel anxious, then you may choose to avoid crowds, like going out on a holiday or shopping during peak times.

Yes, this might be the most natural thing to do, but here's the problem. The problem is that avoidance increases or intensifies anxiety. You may not realize it, but when you avoid something because of fear, the relief of not having to deal with your fear is your biggest reward. And it's addictive too. So, if this time you feared large crowds, by avoiding the fear, you decreased your threshold to that fear.

And because it gave you an instant reward, you're more likely to avoid it again. If large crowds make you uncomfortable, soon smaller crowds will begin to do the same. And with time, your avoidance will push you to a point where the mere sight of people or thought of engaging in the slightest conversation might put you through a panic attack. Identifying and acting against your fears will help you overcome the fear as well as any anxiety that might have accompanied it. With plenty to benefit, it makes sense that you try.

Worksheet 14 - Identifying Your Fears

To face your fears, you must first know what exactly you fear. What is it that troubles you the most? What accelerates your anxiety?

- Reflect on your top five fears - the ones that are coming in the way of your goals and the ones you want to do something about.

- Where do they come from? What are the situations and events that bring on these fears?

- What's the worst that can happen? Imagine them. Describe it in words

- Take your time and don't rush through the experience.

- Review your answers when you are ready.

Acting against Your Fears

Congratulations. You've completed the first step. You're doing great. Now that you've zeroed in on your fears and where they come from, you can create a plan to overcome them.

Worksheet 15 - Taking the Step-Up Approach

- Pick the least feared item from your checklist.
- Create steps that will help you overcome your fear. For instance, Jason fears crowded places (especially malls) and so his steps might include:

Imagining waiting in line at the post office and interacting with people. Going to the post office by himself. Greeting the person at the counter.
Imagining watching a movie at the theatre. Attending a movie with a friend during the weekday, and in time, during the weekend.
Imagining buying groceries from a store. Going grocery shopping all by himself on a weekend. Checking for offers. Spending time at the store.
Imagining visiting a mall during a holiday. Visiting and spending time at the mall before it opens. Visiting and spending time at the mall with a friend when it is open. Visiting and spending time at the mall all by himself during a holiday.

- Take time to reflect on your plan. Keep it real and in order.
- Take time to execute your plan and face your fear, tracking your progress until the fear doesn't bother you anymore.
- Again, don't rush and take your time to live-in the experience. Embrace the changes that come with it.

Begin the Process

Create and Execute Your Plan

Great, so you've tapped into your strengths, recognize what you want and have laid out goals that will keep you busy. What next?

Well, you create a formidable plan to materialize those deliverables.

Your ability to set up a quick, direct and foolproof action plan for your goals is what is going to see you through the finish line. If you walk into the game with just the right cards in your pocket, you've got yourself a winner at the very beginning.

Consider Every Aspect That Might Influence, Conflict or Jeopardize Your Plan

Brainstorm on a properly written plan that lists out specific details of your action steps and deadlines. There is nothing such as an ideal plan. Your plan is only as good as your thoughts are today.

The more you learn, the more your plan is likely to change. Take time to prioritize your action steps and the sequence they are likely to follow. Treat it as the blueprint of your road to success. The more groundwork you invest in it, the more fool-proof and success-oriented it becomes.

Be Mindful of Any possible Setbacks, But Don't Let Them Wear You Down

What if an old fear comes back? What if the anxiety comes back? Will they come back?

Truth is, we don't know. Each person's anxiety and experience are different. They might, but even if they do, you now know how to get on top of them. Don't let the fear of evoking a fear drain you out. You have better things to focus on. Stay positive. You've got this.

No Need to Hurry

Remember-while this might be about achieving your goals, it is also about overcoming your anxiety. You do not want to create a situation where you've taken more than you can chew. You're in this for a lifetime, it's always going to be work-in-progress. But each day, you're better than what you were yesterday.

Know When You've Tried Too Long

Because anxiety forces your thought process to be rigid, it can sometimes make you persist on tasks even when you know they aren't working out. Recognize the signs that you need to stop persisting.

It's Okay to Fall. Fail Too

No one is perfect and there is no ideal plan. Keep asking yourself what's working and what's not? If you think you're missing the bus and there's scope for improvement, don't be ashamed to get back to the drawing board and start over again. You'll be surprised by the wave of new ideas coming your way.

Realign Your Plan. Improvise Too

Always ask yourself, "Is there a better way around?" When you stay open to new ideas, you leave room for creativity and growth.

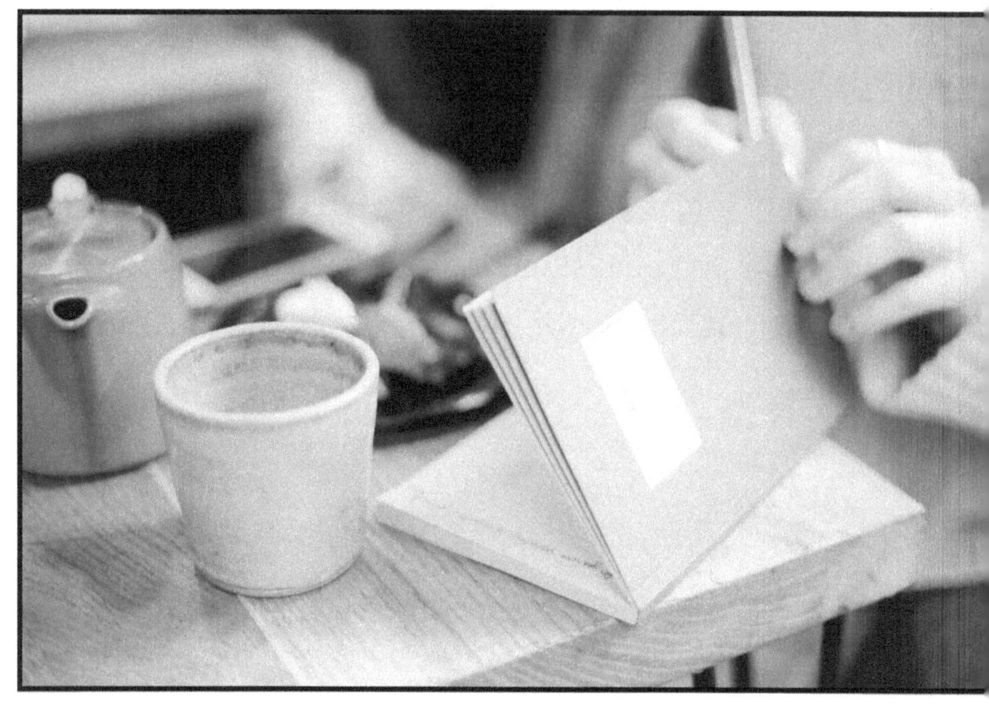

Complete What You've Taken

Uncertainty can trigger a degree of anxiety in most people. But for a person suffering from anxiety, any sense of uncertainty, whether it comes from a space of unfinished tasks or repeated failures, can trigger the worst symptoms. Your anxious mind is probably waiting for a chance to bounce back in and take control. And it will try to do so.

The key is to be aware of this, but not get perturbed by it. Complete what you've taken and only move ahead when you've finished your previous task. The joy of seeing through a project from start to end will give you the confidence to win over anxiety for good.

Become a Better Version of You

Once you've created your plan and find it executing rather well, it's time you reach out for brighter and more rewarding pastures. You've worked hard to make it so far, now, it's time to capitalize on your achievements and make advancements. Experiment ideas and invent them too. Be a game-changer. When you've channelized your energies in the right place and know you have things going for you, you'll leave no room for anxiety or fear to enter your life.

6

NAVIGATING SELF-IMPOSED OBSTACLES

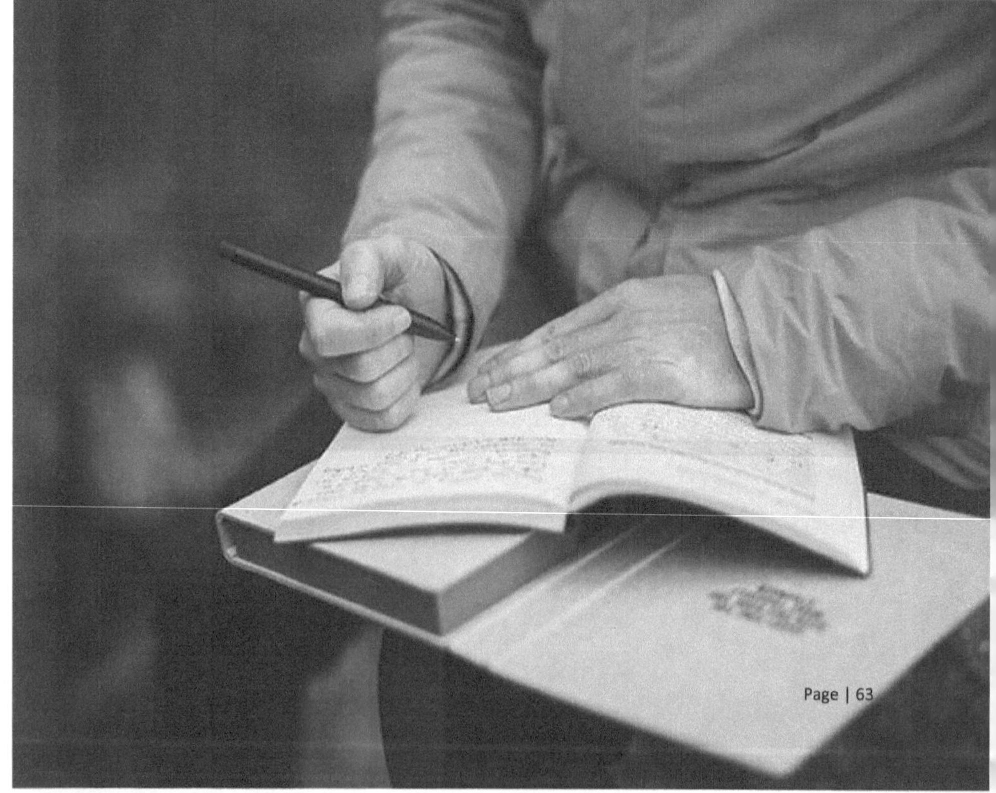

Chapter 6 - Navigating Self-Imposed Obstacles: How to Stop Being a Hard Task Master

The general perception is that people with anxiety live too far in the future. They worry about what might happen the next moment, the next day, next week, next year, but struggle to stay in the present. They fear the unknown and so spend a large part of their time searching from cues from the future.

While this is true, it doesn't quite paint the entire picture. Anxiety can certainly be caused when one anticipates the possibility of facing their fears in the future. But where did these fears come from? Certainly, the origins of it might have stemmed from the person's past.

Moving Ahead of Any past Pain Memories

When something unpleasant happens to you, it is only natural to do everything you can to avoid going it again. Outwardly, this makes sense, and it is healthy to learn from our experiences (good or bad) and move on.

But what happens when you can't move on? What if you become so consumed by the possibility of facing that experience (which might have become a fear or phobia in time) that you become paralyzed by it? What if in the act of moving on, you've dug yourself a grave out of which you cannot come out or live in? What do you do then?

You must face your past to face your fears and make peace with them. To overcome your anxiety for today and tomorrow, it is important that you first heal your past.

Worksheet 16 - Assessing Any past Pain Memories

Chose the most suitable answer.

How do you react when you remember memories from your past that might indicate any prior failure/bad experience/embarrassment/and or sorrow?

- The thought doesn't bother you because you've moved on. You focus on the task ahead.

- You flinch while thinking about the unpleasant experience. Avoid things that could bring back those memories. It does affect your mood, but you can bounce back after some time.

- The thought of these experiences can bring back the worst symptoms of anxiety. You are unable to focus on the task ahead and feel miserable for a long time. The thought never leaves and is always lurking around in the corner of your mind.

If remembering your past is doing you more harm than good, then it's time you leave it behind and move on.

Moving Away from the Past You Need to Leave Behind

Worksheet 17 - Letting Go

Re-visit the past if you can learn from your experiences, but don't engage with it.

Ask yourself:

- What happened? Probe only on the facts.
- What emotions do I feel?
- How can I use this to empower myself and my feelings?
- Is there something I want to express?
- Take responsibility. Focus on healing and moving to a better place.
- How can I heal? What do I need to do to forgive, forget, disconnect, and move on?
- Write down your thoughts. Work on them too.
- Revisit this exercise whenever the feelings return and until you've moved on.
- Make beautiful new memories in place of them.

Overcoming Obsessions

Obsessions are repeated unwelcome thoughts, images or impulses that force a person to act on them. These thoughts can soon become the reason you worry all the time, in turn, creating a breeding ground for your anxiety.

Some obsessions can be harmless at first thought (such as worrying about the tidiness of your house, keeping things in their places, locking doors, switching off appliances), but because these thoughts translate to continuous doubt and worry, they can put a lot of stress on the person experiencing them.

Some thoughts can take a more sinister form (such as harming someone you love, engaging in shameful sexual behaviors and violating another person's dignity). Sadly, compulsions are undesired actions that people repeatedly find themselves doing. They have little control over what happens between thought and action but might have to live with the guilt of their actions forever.

Knowing When You Need Help

Plenty of people experience minor obsessions in one form or the other and that's completely ok. Obsessions might cause no problem. But if your repeated thoughts and actions begin to infringe/violate on yours and society's belief systems, then it can become a serious problem. We suggest you seek medical help then.

Obsessive-Compulsive Disorder (OCD) can cause a great deal of emotional discomfort. It can also consume a considerable amount of time of the person living with it.

Worksheet 18 - Recognizing Any Obsessions

Because obsessions mostly start with thoughts and imagery, it makes sense that you identify them through imagination.

Find a comfortable, private place to sit and work through these questions:

- Reflect on whether you have any distressing, obsessive thought or image?
- Write them down (if any). Visualize them.

- Do they interfere with your peace?
- Do they cause and add to your anxiety?
- Are they harmful by nature?
- How upset do they make you feel?
- Would you rather not think/do what you do as a result of these thoughts?
- Do you want to move to a better place?

Worksheet 19 - Minding Any Obsessions/Compulsions

- Sit with your feelings, gradually telling yourself you can overcome these thoughts and any unfavorable things they might make you do.
- Imagine yourself doing the positive things you want to replace your thoughts/actions with.
- Repeat the thought or image, replaying it several times over (yes, in a compulsive sort of way).
- Continue this imagery for as long as you want or until you feel like you've done a degree of what you wanted to do.
- Repeat this exercise every day, mindfully replacing any negative/unfavorable obsessions with positive imagery that makes you feel good and can set you free.

New Beginnings

Love yourself and feel good about everything you are going to do in the future. The happier and more content you stay within yourself, the more your brain recognizes your happiness to stay away from any unpleasant obsessions/compulsions as a reward. Also, you are likely to feel less anxious too.

Focus on the Positives

Remember that every mistake made is a lesson well-learnt. Take the positives out of the outcome and push further. Staying motivated is all about staying positive and optimistic. Draw inspiration from people who've made a difference in your life. Read plenty and draw inspiration from other achievers.

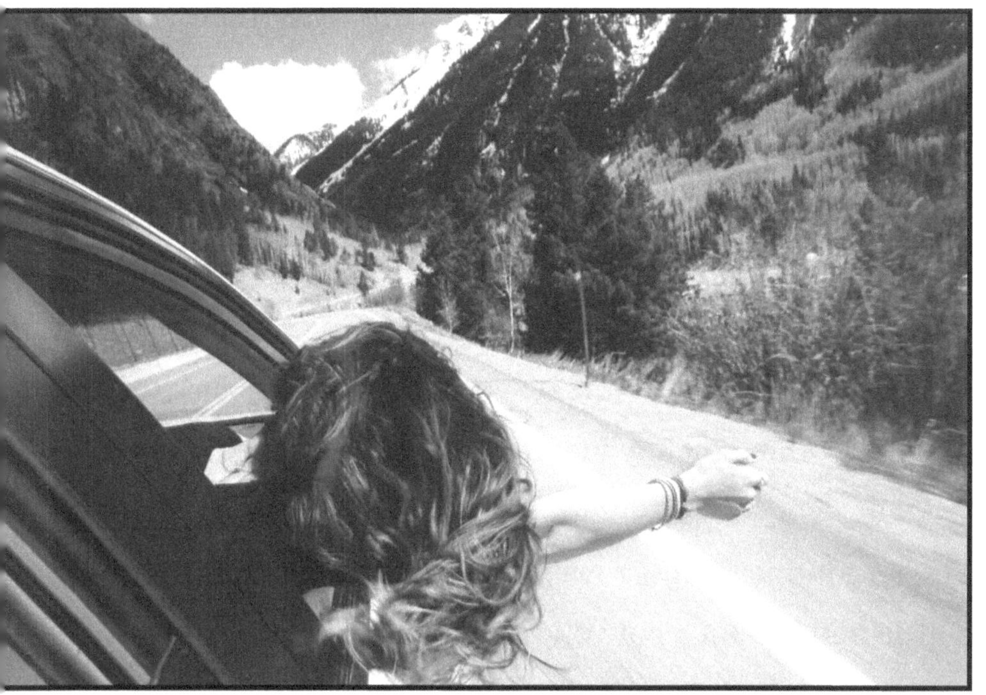

Worksheet 20 – Creating Tomorrow

- Take some time to reflect on how you want you near future to be, starting tomorrow.
- Write them down.
- What obsessions/compulsions do you need/want to start working on immediately?
- How do you plan to approach them?
- Make a mental note of everything you need to face this situation.
- Do you have everything you need?

- Now imagine yourself going through these situations tomorrow.
- Imagine yourself delaying the urge to act on any unfavorable thoughts.
- How far did you go?
- Continue this exercise every day, delaying the urge to act until you don't feel like acting on your impulses because they either don't bother you any more or simply don't exist.

You've got this. Tomorrow is a new beginning. Make it count. Be a little better than what you were today.

7

PREVENTING BURNOUT

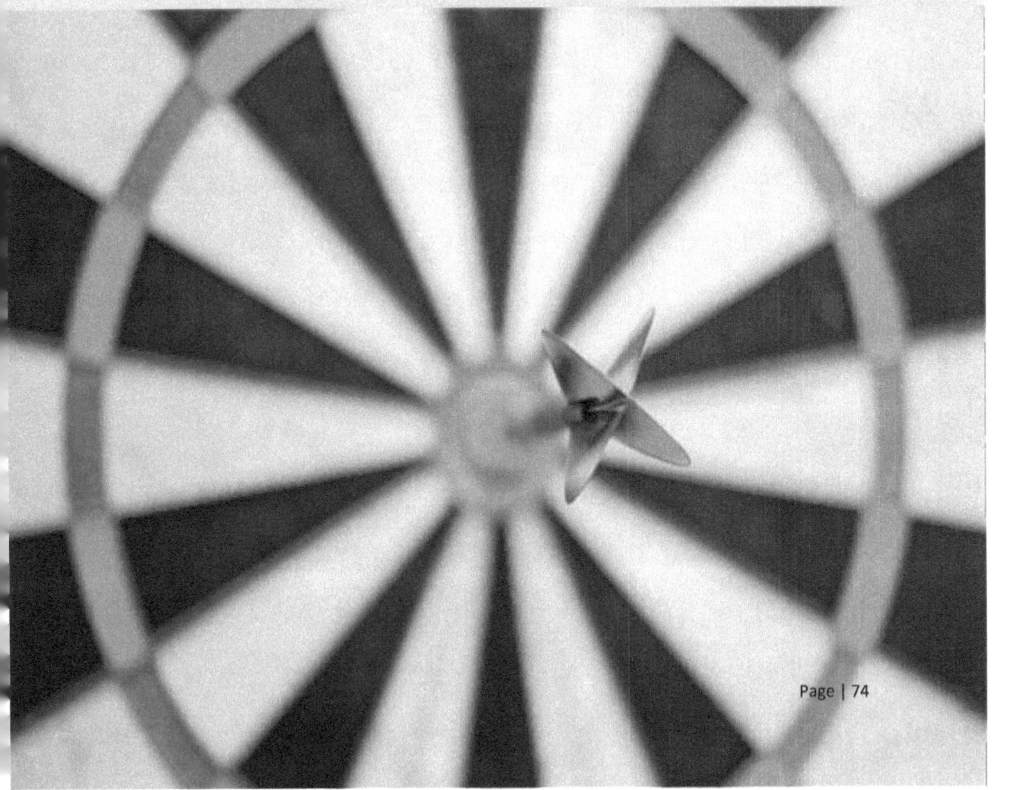

Chapter 7 - Preventing Burnout: How to Overcome Your Anxiety without Getting Tied-Down by the Idea of Perfection

Setting Real Expectations

So, you've understood the origins of your anxiety and are working on your goals. You're also in the process of working on any obsessions and stuck points you might have to come across in the way. The ideal scenario is that you enjoy your progress and learn from any lessons and setbacks. You take everything in stride and don't get too influenced by it.

But sometimes, this can be easier said than done, especially for a person dealing with anxiety. Sometimes, their anxiety-driven expectations can get in the way. This chapter will show you how to focus on the bigger picture. It will show you how to move past any unhelpful standards of perfectionism and be your only competitor because you don't need to compete with anyone but yourself. Being a little better than yesterday, every day, will get you where you want to be without the stress.

Worksheet 21 – Expectation Tracker

Take the below quiz choosing between often, sometimes, and never.

1. How often are you bothered by fears of not measuring up?
2. How often are you bothered by what others will think?
3. How often do you compare yourself with others?
4. How often do you become frustrated with the pace of your success?

Choose the most applicable answer for the below questions:

5. What's your reaction when your friends/colleagues perform better than you?
- You don't panic, take it as healthy competition and work harder
- You start comparing and get anxious with the notion of not being good enough

- You feel miserable and like a failure. You're also anxious for long.

6. On what basis do you set/measure goals and success?

- On personal beliefs and interests
- On borrowed, societal, or other's definitions

7. Do you jump from one unfinished project to another unfinished project when you are anxious or in self-doubt?

- Yes, I cannot concentrate and so try different things.
- Sometimes
- No, I try and work on one thing at a time
- Yes, I have plenty of unfinished projects

Reflect on the answers. They can tell you if your idea of achievement is yours to chase, if it is causing your anxiety, and if you need to alter the course of what you believe is your destination.

Perfectionism and Borrowed Expectations

Setting expectations while chasing goals is a great way to ensure you complete everything that you've set forth for yourself. But if those expectations aren't stemming from your needs, and are, on the contrary, based on what others believe is right, then you're more likely to be living someone else's life. The dreams aren't yours and the pursuit, although committed by you, may feel disconnected in some way. Finally, the success (if you manage the conviction to get there) won't be rewarding enough.

Leaving No Room to Pause. Falter Too

As a result, you may end up feeling that you haven't done enough, aren't good enough. You're likely to work harder, chase farther, with no room to pause. Falter too. You'll always want to feel more because everything that you feel in your pursuit of living other's dreams may not mean as much to you. Unrealistic and borrowed expectations is considered a risk factor for developing anxiety problems. Not every anxious person lives on perfectionism and borrowed dreams, but if you do, then this chapter is for you.

Avoiding Comparisons

A common obstacle while making personal and transformative changes is social comparison. You cannot compare yourself to others when it comes to creating an agenda that works for you (well, you can, but it won't be helpful). A schedule that feels convenient and right for someone else might not be right for you.

Worksheet 22 - Becoming the Change You Want to See

Take time to reflect on your ideals- things that you connect with and things that you want to invite into your life.

How close is it from your current reality?
If it is in alignment, then you can skip this step. But if what you envisioned is a stark contrast to what you're living, then it's time to change the trajectory of your pursuit. It's time to align it to things that resonate with you. Because when you walk this new path that you're about to create, you'll discover your purpose.

And what better way than to live your life with purpose?

Change Everything If You Have To, but Change Them One Thing at a Time

Changes in how you feel are going to come from making a mixture of external changes (such as changes in how you spend your time) and internal changes (such as what you think and believe).

- Reflect on your narrative. What part of it do you need to change?
- What do you need to do to act out the change?
- Make a list of steps to get there.
- Start working on them, one step at a time.

Fear of Feedback

At large, feedback endorses progress. Used constructively, it can help people improve. However, that might not necessarily be the case all the time or for all people, especially anxious people. Anxious people mostly avoid it because of the additional layer of expectation and criticism it can put on them. Most anxious people already feel stifled by all their compulsions, obsessions, expectations, perfectionism. Another lay may not help. Here's how you can manage feedback and use it constructively.

Worksheet 23 - Overcoming Feedback Fears

Think of a situation in your life that you know will benefit from feedback, but you're avoiding it. Ask yourself:

- Why am I avoiding this feedback when I know it might be helpful?
- How likely does it feel that I'm going to get very negative feedback?
- How close is it to the truth?

Ok, you now know that already. Now ask yourself:
- How will I benefit from this feedback?
- What's the worst that can happen?
- Does it measure up to the possible benefits?
- Do I assistance to cope with any resulting emotions? For instance, you might want to talk to a friend.

Finally, if the feedback is going to be beneficial. Prepare to receive it.

- Think of one specific instance in the past when feedback (negative feedback because that's what you mostly fear) was very helpful to you.
- Factor any chances of bias/hostile feedback
- Recognize their signs and know when to not take them seriously
- Invite the experience knowing that you've got yourself covered whatever may be the outcome.

Reward Yourself. You've Made Great Progress

After you've worked on a task you've been avoiding, allow yourself to enjoy the fruits of your labor by taking time to appreciate yourself, doing something you like to do. Choose rewards that can help you progress from where you are.

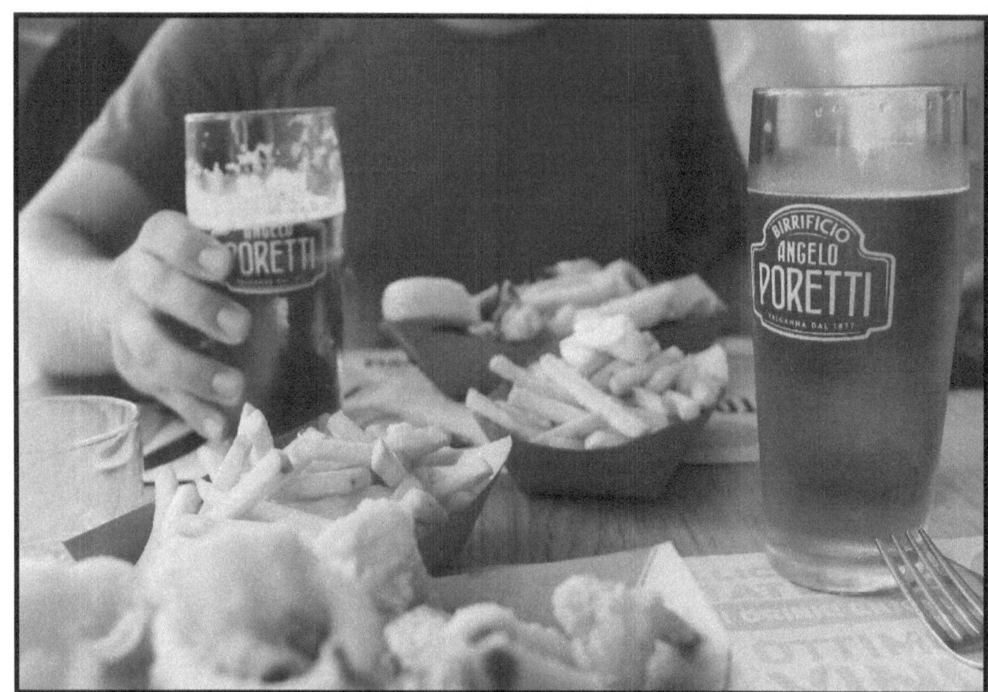

Rewarding yourself with a supersize portion of fries while on a weight loss journey won't help. Instead, pick up something that you always wanted to wear, only in one size lesser. Not only will this motivate you to reach the next milestone, but you'll also know that you have a nice little reward waiting for you when you get there.

CHAPTER 8

HOW TO BANISH WORRY AND LIVE PANIC-FREE

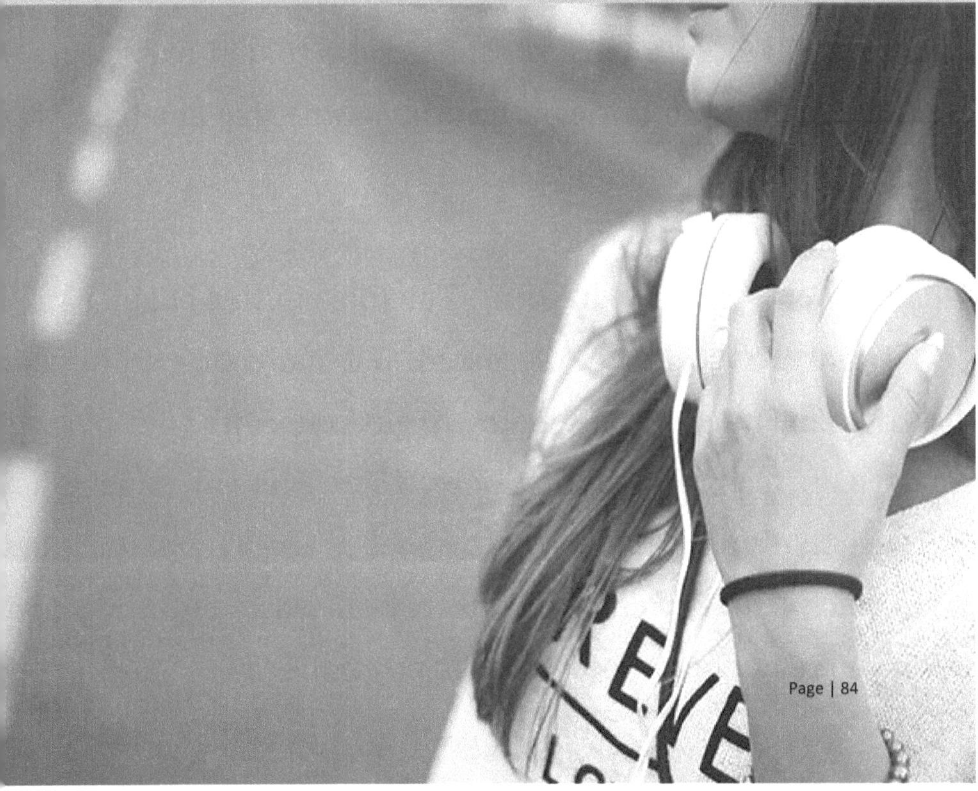

Chapter 8 - You've Got This: How to Banish Worry and Live Panic-Free

You've done a great job moving into the final chapter. We are very happy for you.

We've covered many different topics throughout this; from topics that help you understand your anxiety to ones that help overcome it and move to a place of acceptance and peace. Each chapter is filled with purposeful worksheets that are specially designed to take you through the process one step at a time, at a pace that is convenient for you.

This chapter is slightly different. The tools in this chapter rally on all that we've already discussed, but more practically and directly. This time, it is intending to gift you a quick lift of sorts when you're feeling low and anxious. There isn't any explanation (because that's what the rest of the book is about). But there are some quick-fixes and effective tips that can get you up and about when you're not quite your usual-happy self.

Simplify

If you've been practicing the worksheets presented in this book, you might have a better idea of how your anxiety plays out. You might also know the handful of issues that trouble you - the ones that still creep up on you when you least expect them to. Here are some quick, but effective tips to keep them down and out of your way for longer periods.

Anti-Anxiety Formulas

Breathe

When you're anxious, your mind can get caught up battling the thoughts ringing its head. You can become so consumed by the process of balancing your emotions that you fail to recognize the physical effects of it. There are some tell-tale signs which when addressed can instantly help bring down your anxiety. Your breathing is at the top of that list.

Typically, when anxious, your breathing quickens and becomes shallow. This goes against the natural pattern of breathing which is slow and deep. And because our lives depend on our breath, any deviance in this pattern can add to your stress and make you more uncomfortable. You can quickly counter this by focusing on your breath:

1. Place one hand on your abdomen and the other on your chest.
2. Breathe in slowly, focusing on expanding your abdomen first and then your chest.
3. Exhale slowly, telling yourself to relax when you breathe out.
4. Repeat Steps 1 through 3 for at least ten breaths.

Exercise

Your body is not meant to be stressed. It's meant to be happy, healthy, and at peace. And so, when you get upset, your body is alarmed and responds by producing stress hormones. Exercise has proved to be very effective in burning these hormones.

Exercises such as running, jogging, brisk walking, and/or aerobics for as little as 15 to 20 minutes, at a time when you're stressed, can do wonders to alleviate symptoms of anxiety. Choose any physical activity that you enjoy doing. The fact that you also like what you're doing will help shift you to a happier and stress-free phase.

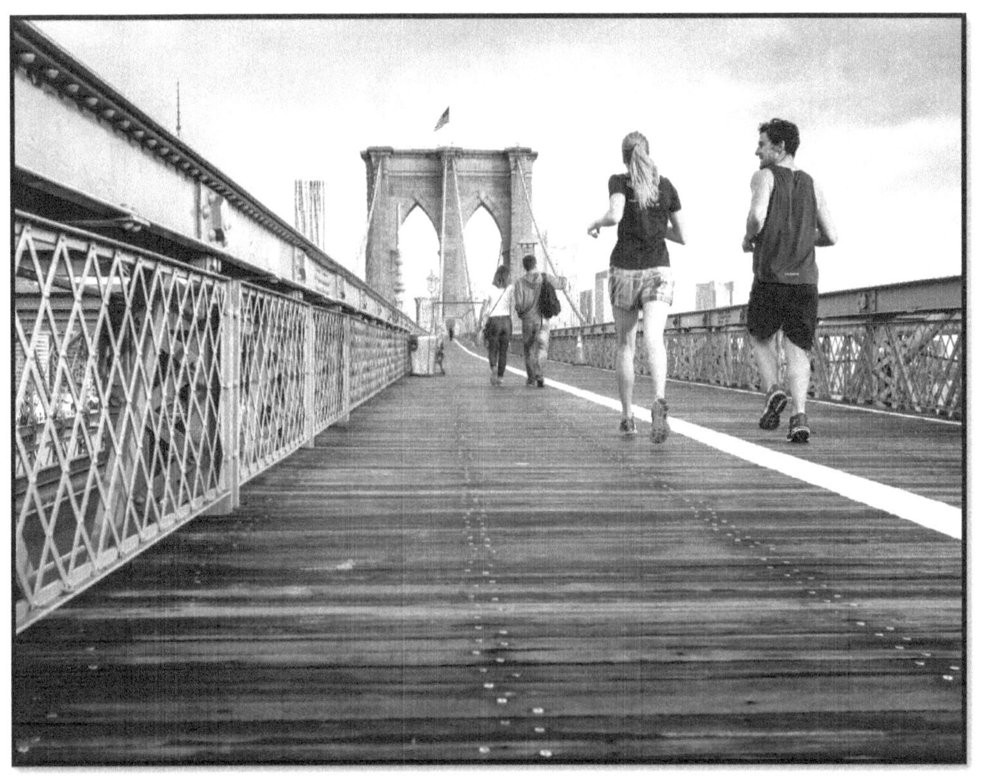

Express Yourself. Talk It Out or Journal Your Thoughts

We are social creatures. We want to mingle and thrive as a collective society. And so, by this nature, it is natural for you to feel better when you connect with or talk to someone you understand and who understands you.

Rally your support system. Call a loved one and talk about what's troubling you. Even if you're somebody who doesn't like to mingle a lot, you might find it helpful to just let things out of your system. If you don't have anyone you can immediately call and talk to, try and journal your thoughts.

Do not hesitate to talk to yourself either. Try and understand exactly what's bothering you and the best way to do that is to ask yourself questions.

- What's bothering me?
- Does my narrative sound correct?
- Is there another way of looking at what happened?
- How can shift to a better place?

Always ask yourself questions because when you do, you may get vital information that can then stimulate your thinking further, perhaps from an all new reasonable and refreshing angle.

Listen to Music

Sound stimulates the mind and body. It can inspire you or upset you. When you're upset, try and listen to music that soothes your mind. Listen to whatever makes you happy.

Spend Time with Pets

Studies prove that spending time with pets promotes better moods and health. Spend time with your pets, play with them too. You'll quickly realize your anxiety disappearing away.

Give Your Mind Something More Productive to Chew On

Often, when you're stressed, your mind refuses to think outside the situation. It focuses on the discomfort and replays the events that led to it several times over. If the worry is serious and needs assistance, then we urge you to consult a therapist. But if it's more minor in intensity and caution, then we recommend distracting it with some of your favorite activities.

Try:

- Reading a good novel
- Watching a movie
- Playing a sport
- Spending time with family
- Walking your pet
- And anything else that makes you happy

Stay in the Present

Remember that most of what has upset you has happened in the past. The moment has passed. And a lot of what you may worry about may be in the future. They happened yet and might never happen too. Instead of toggling between the past and future, stay in the present. Notice your breath because that's living in the present. Focus on your breath as mentioned before and bring yourself back to the present.

Your Anxiety Your Journey

As you progress further, you'll gain a deeper understanding of the origins of your anxiety, you'll also discover ways to manage and overcome them. At this point, we urge you to take a moment to pause and reflect on everything you've learned about yourself so far. It can get overwhelming and we want you to know that that's completely expected and normal.

You Decide. Ready or Not?

You've made great progress and we are very happy that we can be a part of it. At the same time, we want you to also know that this journey is yours to take. Reflect and conclude on what's right for you and what's not. Don't rush into things. Instead, take time to regroup and recalibrate. If you wish, take time off to think about your journey till now, practice everything that you've learned so far. You decide when and how you want to move things ahead.

This book is filled with plenty of practical tools to help address your anxiety. Take time to truly work on it because when you do, you'll be rewarded with lifelong benefits.

Finally, reflect on everything that's been shared with you through this book and figure out what works for you

Worksheet 24 - Gathering Your Tools

- Take a few moments to reflect on how the various systems in this chapter have worked for you.
- Make a note of the techniques that worked for you. Feel free to improvise and make them yours.

Conclusion

This is the end of our journey together for now. Thank you for the effort you've put into practicing and understanding the many concepts mentioned in this book. We hope you've learned of ways to manage your anxiety, and in time, overcome it.

At this point, we urge you to keep referring to your notes, to keep working on the many practice exercises provided. As you progress further and sharpen your understanding, you'll develop skills that can help you arise above all anxious periods.

Best wishes.

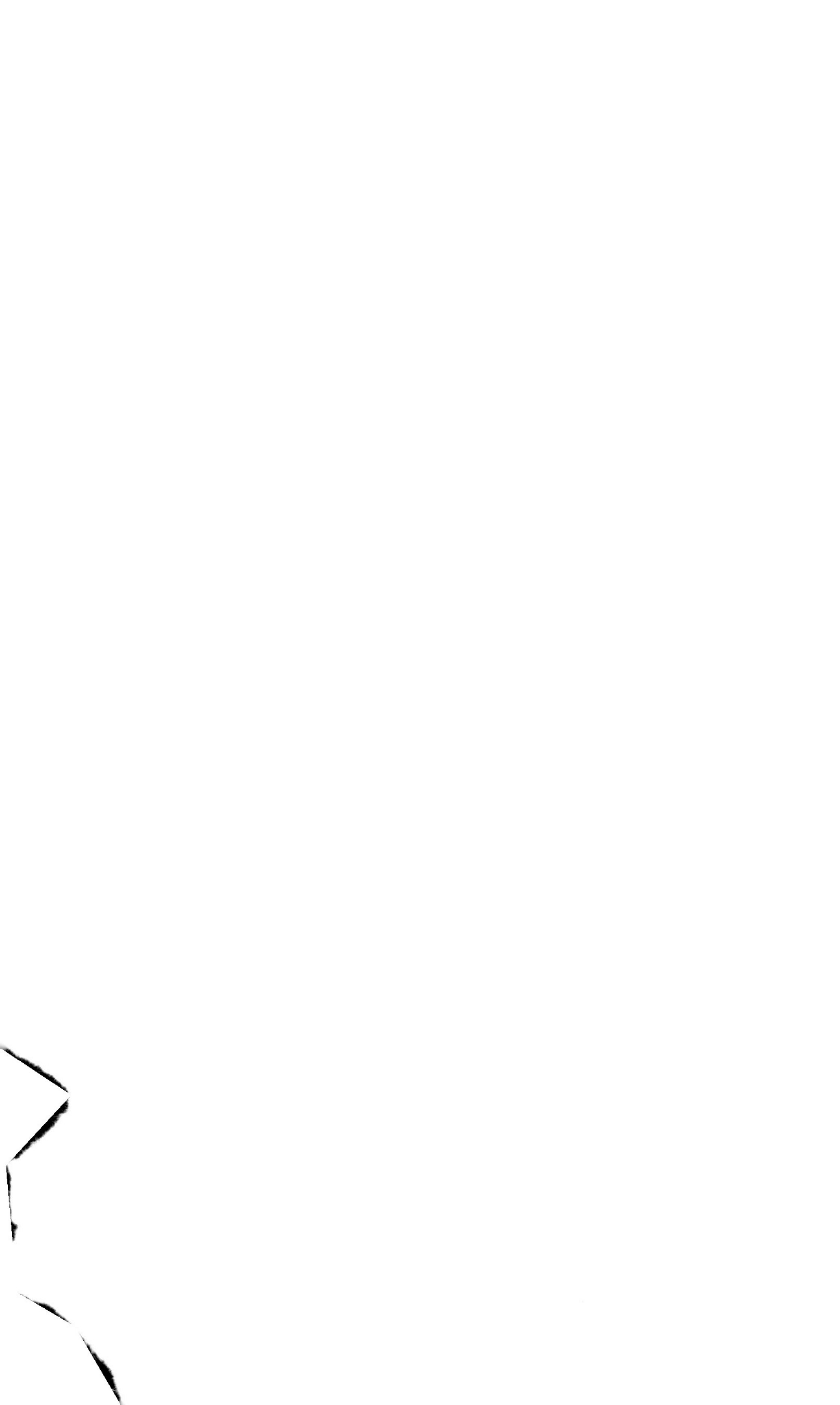